LOW-CALORIE MEAL PREP FOR BEGINNERS

Easy, Healthy Recipes to Help You Lose Weight

Dr Lily Morgan

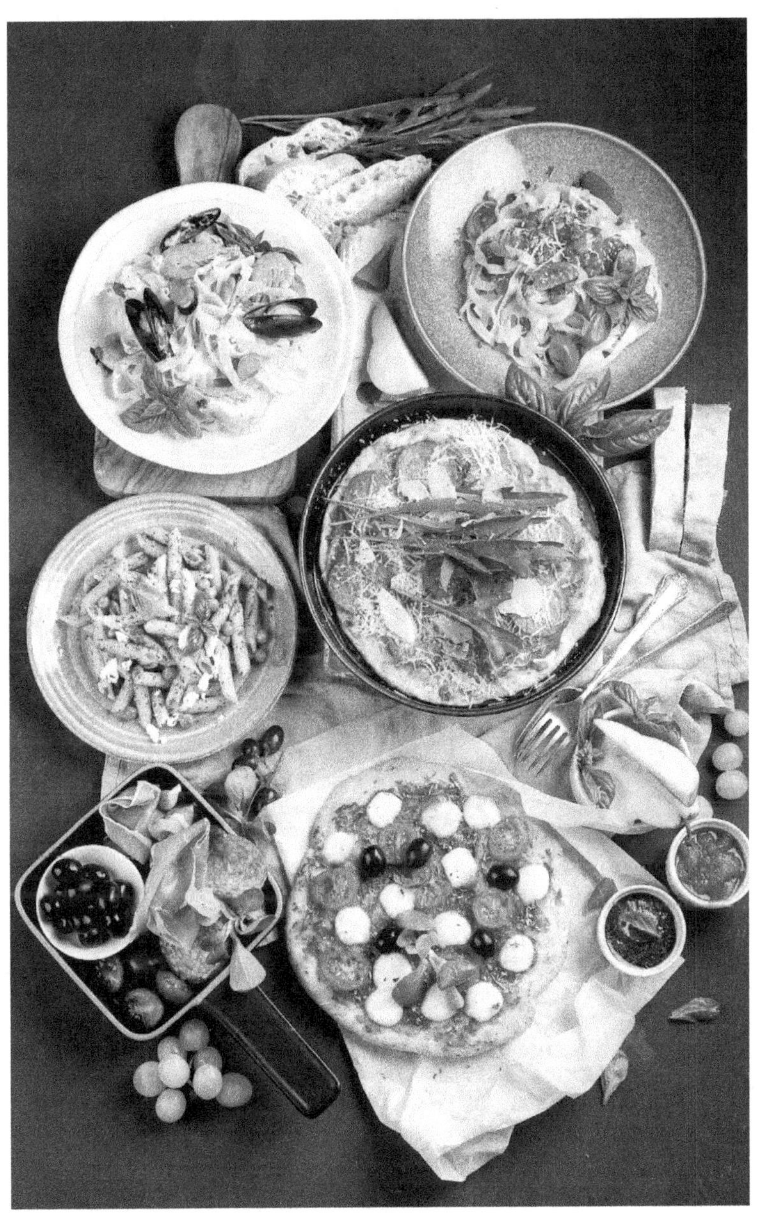

TABLE OF CONTENTS

Chapter 5: Snacks and Appetizers 63

INTRODUCTION

In today's fast-paced world, understanding the nuances of low-calorie meal preparation is more crucial than ever. Low-calorie meal prep is not just about counting calories; it's a holistic approach to nourishing your body while managing your weight. Let's delve into the core concepts.

Understanding Low-Calorie Meal Prep:

Low-calorie meal prep is a deliberate and thoughtful way of planning and preparing meals with a focus on reducing caloric intake without sacrificing nutritional value. It's not about deprivation; rather, it's about making informed choices to create balanced, satisfying meals that align with your health goals.

Key aspects of understanding low-calorie meal prep include:

1. **Portion Control:** Controlling portion sizes is fundamental. Smaller portions help reduce overall

calorie consumption, while ensuring you still enjoy your favorite foods.

2. **Nutrient Density**: Low-calorie meals should be nutrient-dense, providing essential vitamins and minerals without excess calories. This means emphasizing fruits, vegetables, lean proteins, and whole grains.

3. **Balanced Macronutrients**: Focus on the right balance of macronutrients - carbohydrates, proteins, and healthy fats. This balance supports energy levels, muscle maintenance, and overall well-being.

4. **Mindful Cooking Techniques**: Techniques like grilling, roasting, steaming, and sautéing with minimal oil help reduce calorie content while retaining flavor.

5. **Meal Planning:** Plan your meals in advance to avoid impulsive, calorie-laden choices. A well-structured meal plan can be your best ally in low-calorie meal prep.

Benefits of Low-Calorie Eating:

Embracing a low-calorie eating approach offers a plethora of benefits that go beyond weight management:

1. **Weight Control**: The most apparent benefit is weight management. Consuming fewer calories than you burn results in weight loss, making it an effective strategy for those aiming to shed extra pounds.

2. **Improved Health**: Low-calorie diets are associated with lower risk factors for chronic diseases such as heart disease, diabetes, and hypertension. They can help improve overall health and reduce the strain on vital organs.

3. **Enhanced Energy:** Balanced low-calorie meals provide a sustained source of energy without the highs and crashes associated with high-calorie, high-sugar foods.

4. **Mental Clarity:** Low-calorie eating can lead to improved cognitive function, as it reduces inflammation and oxidative stress that can affect brain health.

5. **Better Digestion:** Nutrient-dense, low-calorie foods are often easier to digest, leading to better gut health and enhanced nutrient absorption.

6. **Longevity**: Some studies suggest that low-calorie eating might extend lifespan by reducing the risk of age-related diseases.

In summary, understanding low-calorie meal prep and the benefits of low-calorie eating is not about adopting a restrictive lifestyle. It's about making conscious, healthful choices that can lead to a more vibrant and fulfilling life. By focusing on nutrient density, portion control, and balanced meals, you can embark on a journey towards better health and overall well-being.

Chapter 1: 30 Day Meal Plan

Week 1

Day 1

- Breakfast: Scrambled Egg Whites with Spinach
- Lunch: Grilled Chicken Salad
- Dinner: Baked Salmon with Asparagus
- Snacks: Guacamole and Veggie Sticks
- Dessert: Berry Parfait

Day 2

- Breakfast: Overnight Oats with Fresh Berries
- Lunch: Quinoa and Black Bean Bowl
- Dinner: Spaghetti Squash with Marinara
- Snacks: Sliced Cucumber with Hummus
- Dessert: Chocolate Banana Ice Cream

Day 3

- Breakfast: Greek Yogurt Parfait
- Lunch: Turkey and Veggie Wrap
- Dinner: Teriyaki Chicken with Broccoli

- Snacks: Baked Sweet Potato Fries
- Dessert: Baked Apple with Cinnamon

Day 4

- Breakfast: Avocado Toast with Poached Egg
- Lunch: Lentil Soup
- Dinner: Stuffed Bell Peppers
- Snacks: Mixed Nuts
- Dessert: Greek Yogurt Cheesecake

Day 5

- Breakfast: Whole Wheat Pancakes
- Lunch: Caprese Salad
- Dinner: Eggplant Parmesan
- Snacks: Greek Yogurt and Berries
- Dessert: Mango Sorbet

Day 6

- Breakfast: Chia Seed Pudding
- Lunch: Tuna Salad Lettuce Wraps
- Dinner: Lemon Garlic Shrimp and Quinoa
- Snacks: Popcorn

- Dessert: Dark Chocolate-Dipped Strawberries

Day 7

- Breakfast: Veggie Omelette
- Lunch: Zucchini Noodles with Pesto
- Dinner: Turkey and Sweet Potato Chili
- Snacks: Edamame
- Dessert: Mini Fruit Tarts

Week 2

Day 8

- Breakfast: Quinoa Breakfast Bowl
- Lunch: Chicken and Vegetable Stir-Fry
- Dinner: Beef and Broccoli Stir-Fry
- Snacks: Rice Cakes with Peanut Butter
- Dessert: Almond and Coconut Bites

Day 9

- Breakfast: Banana Nut Muffins
- Lunch: Sweet Potato and Chickpea Curry
- Dinner: Butternut Squash Soup
- Snacks: Deviled Eggs

- Dessert: Vanilla Chia Seed Pudding

Day 10

- Breakfast: Breakfast Burrito
- Lunch: Caesar Salad with Grilled Shrimp
- Dinner: Spinach and Feta Stuffed Chicken Breast
- Snacks: Salsa and Baked Tortilla Chips
- Dessert: Mixed Berry Crisp

Day 11

- Breakfast: Cottage Cheese and Fruit Bowl
- Lunch: Hummus and Veggie Wrap
- Dinner: Black Bean and Corn Salad
- Snacks: Cottage Cheese with Pineapple
- Dessert: Lemon Sorbet

Day 12

- Breakfast: Oatmeal with Almond Butter
- Lunch: Cucumber and Feta Salad
- Dinner: Grilled Portobello Mushrooms
- Snacks: Spinach and Artichoke Dip
- Dessert: Chocolate Protein Balls

Day 13

- Breakfast: Sweet Potato Hash
- Lunch: Spinach and Mushroom Quesadilla
- Dinner: Veggie Stir-Fried Rice
- Snacks: Trail Mix
- Dessert: Rice Pudding

Day 14

- Breakfast: Protein-Packed Smoothie
- Lunch: Couscous and Veggie Bowl
- Dinner: Baked Cod with Lemon Dill Sauce
- Snacks: Stuffed Mushrooms
- Dessert: Frozen Grapes

Week 3

Day 15

- Breakfast: Scrambled Egg Whites with Spinach
- Lunch: Grilled Chicken Salad
- Dinner: Baked Salmon with Asparagus
- Snacks: Guacamole and Veggie Sticks
- Dessert: Berry Parfait

Day 16

- Breakfast: Overnight Oats with Fresh Berries
- Lunch: Quinoa and Black Bean Bowl
- Dinner: Spaghetti Squash with Marinara
- Snacks: Sliced Cucumber with Hummus
- Dessert: Chocolate Banana Ice Cream

Day 17

- Break Breakfast: Greek Yogurt Parfait
- Lunch: Turkey and Veggie Wrap
- Dinner: Teriyaki Chicken with Broccoli
- Snacks: Baked Sweet Potato Fries
- Dessert: Baked Apple with Cinnamon

Day 18

- Breakfast: Avocado Toast with Poached Egg
- Lunch: Lentil Soup
- Dinner: Stuffed Bell Peppers
- Snacks: Mixed Nuts
- Dessert: Greek Yogurt Cheesecake

Day 19

- Breakfast: Whole Wheat Pancakes
- Lunch: Caprese Salad
- Dinner: Eggplant Parmesan
- Snacks: Greek Yogurt and Berries
- Dessert: Mango Sorbet

Day 20

- Breakfast: Chia Seed Pudding
- Lunch: Tuna Salad Lettuce Wraps
- Dinner: Lemon Garlic Shrimp and Quinoa
- Snacks: Popcorn
- Dessert: Dark Chocolate-Dipped Strawberries

Day 21

- Breakfast: Veggie Omelette
- Lunch: Zucchini Noodles with Pesto
- Dinner: Turkey and Sweet Potato Chili
- Snacks: Edamame
- Dessert: Mini Fruit Tarts

Week 4

Day 22

- Breakfast: Quinoa Breakfast Bowl
- Lunch: Chicken and Vegetable Stir-Fry
- Dinner: Beef and Broccoli Stir-Fry
- Snacks: Rice Cakes with Peanut Butter
- Dessert: Almond and Coconut Bites

Day 23

- Breakfast: Banana Nut Muffins
- Lunch: Sweet Potato and Chickpea Curry
- Dinner: Butternut Squash Soup
- Snacks: Deviled Eggs
- Dessert: Vanilla Chia Seed Pudding

Day 24

- Breakfast: Breakfast Burrito
- Lunch: Caesar Salad with Grilled Shrimp
- Dinner: Spinach and Feta Stuffed Chicken Breast
- Snacks: Salsa and Baked Tortilla Chips
- Dessert: Mixed Berry Crisp

Day 25

- Breakfast: Cottage Cheese and Fruit Bowl
- Lunch: Hummus and Veggie Wrap
- Dinner: Black Bean and Corn Salad
- Snacks: Cottage Cheese with Pineapple
- Dessert: Lemon Sorbet

Day 26

- Breakfast: Oatmeal with Almond Butter
- Lunch: Cucumber and Feta Salad
- Dinner: Grilled Portobello Mushrooms
- Snacks: Spinach and Artichoke Dip
- Dessert: Chocolate Protein Balls

Day 27

- Breakfast: Sweet Potato Hash
- Lunch: Spinach and Mushroom Quesadilla
- Dinner: Veggie Stir-Fried Rice
- Snacks: Trail Mix
- Dessert: Rice Pudding

Day 28

- Breakfast: Protein-Packed Smoothie
- Lunch: Couscous and Veggie Bowl
- Dinner: Baked Cod with Lemon Dill Sauce
- Snacks: Stuffed Mushrooms
- Dessert: Frozen Grapes

Day 29

- Breakfast: Scrambled Egg Whites with Spinach
- Lunch: Grilled Chicken Salad
- Dinner: Baked Salmon with Asparagus
- Snacks: Guacamole and Veggie Sticks
- Dessert: Berry Parfait

Day 30

- Breakfast: Overnight Oats with Fresh Berries
- Lunch: Quinoa and Black Bean Bowl
- Dinner: Spaghetti Squash with Marinara
- Snacks: Sliced Cucumber with Hummus
- Dessert: Chocolate Banana Ice Cream

Congratulations on completing your 30-day low-calorie meal plan! This plan has provided you with a variety of nutritious and delicious meals for an entire month. You can continue to use and modify these recipes to maintain a healthy eating lifestyle. Enjoy your journey to better health!

Chapter 2: Breakfast Recipes

In this chapter, we'll explore delicious and nutritious breakfast recipes that are perfect for those on a low-calorie journey. Whether you prefer something savory or sweet, there's a recipe here to satisfy your taste buds. Let's dive into these mouthwatering options:

Scrambled Egg Whites with Spinach

Ingredients:

- 4 egg whites
- A handful of fresh spinach
- Salt and pepper to taste

Instructions:

1. Whisk the egg whites in a bowl.
2. Heat a non-stick pan and add the egg whites.
3. Add spinach and cook until the eggs are set.
4. Season with salt and pepper.

Overnight Oats with Fresh Berries

Ingredients:

- 1/2 cup rolled oats
- 1 cup unsweetened almond milk
- 1/2 cup fresh berries (strawberries, blueberries, or raspberries)
- 1 tablespoon honey (optional)

Instructions:

1. In a jar, combine oats and almond milk.
2. Add berries and honey (if desired).
3. Seal the jar and refrigerate overnight.
4. Enjoy your ready-to-eat breakfast in the morning.

Greek Yogurt Parfait

Ingredients:

- 1 cup Greek yogurt
- 1/2 cup granola
- 1/2 cup mixed berries (blueberries, strawberries, and raspberries)

Instructions:

1. In a glass, layer Greek yogurt, granola, and berries.
2. Repeat the layers.
3. Top with a few extra berries.

Avocado Toast with Poached Egg

Ingredients:

*   1 slice whole wheat bread
*   1/2 ripe avocado
*   1 poached egg
*   Salt and pepper

Instructions:

1. Toast the whole wheat bread.
2. Mash the avocado and spread it on the toast.
3. Top with a poached egg.
4. Season with salt and pepper.

Whole Wheat Pancakes

Ingredients:

*   1 cup whole wheat flour

- 1 tablespoon honey

- 1 teaspoon baking powder

- 1 cup almond milk

- 1 egg

- 1/2 teaspoon vanilla extract

Instructions:

1. In a bowl, mix flour, honey, and baking powder.

2. Add almond milk, egg, and vanilla extract. Mix until smooth.

3. Cook pancakes on a non-stick griddle until golden.

Chia Seed Pudding

Ingredients:

- 2 tablespoons chia seeds

- 1 cup almond milk

- 1/2 teaspoon vanilla extract

- 1 tablespoon maple syrup

- Fresh berries for topping

Instructions:

1. In a jar, combine chia seeds, almond milk, vanilla extract, and maple syrup.

2. Stir well and refrigerate for a few hours or overnight.

3. Top with fresh berries before serving.

Veggie Omelette

Ingredients:

- 2 eggs
- Chopped bell peppers, onions, and tomatoes
- Salt and pepper
- Olive oil for cooking

Instructions:

1. Beat the eggs in a bowl and season with salt and pepper.

2. Heat a non-stick pan with a little olive oil.

3. Add chopped vegetables and sauté until tender.

4. Pour the beaten eggs over the veggies and cook until set.

Green Smoothie Bowl

Ingredients:

- 1 cup spinach
- 1/2 banana
- 1/2 cup unsweetened almond milk
- 1 tablespoon chia seeds
- Toppings: sliced banana, berries, and granola

Instructions:

1. Blend spinach, banana, almond milk, and chia seeds until smooth.
2. Pour the smoothie into a bowl.
3. Add your favorite toppings.

Quinoa Breakfast Bowl

Ingredients:

- 1/2 cup cooked quinoa
- 1/4 cup Greek yogurt
- 1/4 cup mixed nuts and dried fruit
- Honey for drizzling

Instructions:

1. In a bowl, layer quinoa, Greek yogurt, and the nut and fruit mix.

2. Drizzle with honey for sweetness.

Banana Nut Muffins

Ingredients:

- 1 cup mashed ripe bananas
- 1/4 cup unsweetened applesauce
- 1/4 cup honey
- 1 egg
- 1 teaspoon vanilla extract
- 1 cup whole wheat flour
- 1/2 cup chopped nuts
- 1/2 teaspoon baking soda
- 1/2 teaspoon baking powder

Instructions:

1. Preheat your oven to 350°F (175°C).

2. In a bowl, mix mashed bananas, applesauce, honey, egg, and vanilla extract.

3. In another bowl, combine flour, nuts, baking soda, and baking powder.

4. Add the dry ingredients to the wet ingredients and mix until just combined.

5. Pour the batter into muffin cups and bake for 20-25 minutes.

Breakfast Burrito

Ingredients:

- 1 whole wheat tortilla
- Scrambled eggs (2-3 egg whites)
- Sautéed bell peppers and onions
- Salsa for topping

Instructions:

1. Lay the tortilla flat.

2. Add scrambled eggs and sautéed vegetables.

3. Roll it up and top with salsa.

Cottage Cheese and Fruit Bowl

Ingredients:

- 1/2 cup low-fat cottage cheese
- Mixed fresh fruits (berries, pineapple, and melon)
- A drizzle of honey

Instructions:

1. In a bowl, combine cottage cheese and fresh fruits.
2. Drizzle with honey for extra sweetness.

Oatmeal with Almond Butter

Ingredients:

- 1/2 cup rolled oats
- 1 cup almond milk
- 1 tablespoon almond butter
- Sliced bananas for topping

Instructions:

1. Cook oats with almond milk until creamy.
2. Stir in almond butter.
3. Top with sliced bananas.

Sweet Potato Hash

Ingredients:

- 1 sweet potato, diced
- Chopped bell peppers and onions
- Olive oil for cooking
- Seasonings of your choice

Instructions:

1. Heat olive oil in a pan.
2. Add sweet potatoes, bell peppers, and onions.
3. Sauté until sweet potatoes are tender and lightly browned.

Protein-Packed Smoothie

Ingredients:

- 1 scoop of your favorite protein powder
- 1 cup unsweetened almond milk
- 1/2 banana
- Handful of spinach
- Ice cubes

Instructions:

1. Blend all the ingredients until smooth.

2. Enjoy a protein-packed, filling smoothie.

Chapter 3: Lunch Recipes

In this chapter, we'll explore delicious and nutritious lunch recipes that are perfect for your low-calorie meal prep journey. From hearty salads to flavorful wraps and comforting soups, these recipes will make your midday meal a delightful experience. Let's dive into these mouthwatering creations!

Grilled Chicken Salad

Ingredients:

- 2 boneless, skinless chicken breasts
- 1 teaspoon olive oil
- Salt and pepper to taste
- Mixed greens
- Cherry tomatoes
- Cucumber slices
- Red onion rings
- Balsamic vinaigrette

Instructions:

1. Preheat the grill.
2. Brush chicken breasts with olive oil and season with salt and pepper.
3. Grill the chicken for about 6-8 minutes per side or until fully cooked.
4. Slice the grilled chicken into strips.
5. In a large bowl, toss the mixed greens, cherry tomatoes, cucumber slices, and red onion rings.
6. Top the salad with the grilled chicken strips.
7. Drizzle with balsamic vinaigrette and serve.

Quinoa and Black Bean Bowl

Ingredients:

- 1 cup quinoa
- 2 cups vegetable broth
- 1 can of black beans, drained and rinsed
- Corn kernels
- Diced bell peppers
- Chopped cilantro
- Lime juice
- Salt and pepper

Instructions:

1. Rinse quinoa and cook in vegetable broth according to package instructions.
2. In a bowl, combine cooked quinoa, black beans, corn kernels, diced bell peppers, and chopped cilantro.
3. Squeeze fresh lime juice over the mixture and season with salt and pepper.
4. Toss everything together and serve as a hearty bowl.

Turkey and Veggie Wrap

Ingredients:

- Whole wheat tortillas
- Sliced turkey breast
- Hummus
- Sliced cucumber
- Sliced red bell pepper
- Spinach leaves

Instructions:

1. Lay out a whole wheat tortilla.
2. Spread a layer of hummus over the tortilla.

3. Place sliced turkey, cucumber, red bell pepper, and spinach leaves on top.

4. Roll up the tortilla tightly, tucking in the sides.

5. Slice in half and enjoy your delicious turkey and veggie wrap.

Lentil Soup

Ingredients:

- 1 cup dried green or brown lentils
- Chopped onion
- Minced garlic
- Diced carrots
- Diced celery
- Vegetable broth
- Cumin
- Paprika
- Salt and pepper

Instructions:

1. Rinse lentils and set aside.

2. In a large pot, sauté chopped onion and minced garlic until fragrant.

3. Add diced carrots and celery and cook for a few minutes.

4. Pour in vegetable broth and add lentils.

5. Season with cumin, paprika, salt, and pepper.

6. Simmer until lentils and vegetables are tender.

7. Serve this hearty lentil soup hot.

Caprese Salad

Ingredients:

- Fresh tomatoes
- Fresh mozzarella cheese
- Fresh basil leaves
- Balsamic glaze
- Olive oil
- Salt and pepper

Instructions:

1. Slice fresh tomatoes and fresh mozzarella cheese.

2. Arrange the tomato and mozzarella slices on a plate.

3. Tuck fresh basil leaves between the slices.

4. Drizzle with balsamic glaze and olive oil.

5. Season with salt and pepper.

6. Enjoy this classic Caprese salad.

Tuna Salad Lettuce Wraps

Ingredients:

- Canned tuna in water, drained
- Greek yogurt
- Chopped celery
- Chopped red onion
- Diced pickles
- Lettuce leaves
- Dill
- Salt and pepper

Instructions:

1. In a bowl, mix canned tuna, Greek yogurt, chopped celery, chopped red onion, and diced pickles.
2. Season with dill, salt, and pepper.
3. Spoon the tuna salad into lettuce leaves.
4. Roll them up and secure with toothpicks for a satisfying, low-calorie meal.

Zucchini Noodles with Pesto

Ingredients:

- Zucchini noodles
- Homemade or store-bought pesto sauce
- Cherry tomatoes
- Pine nuts
- Parmesan cheese

Instructions:

1. Spiralize zucchini into noodle-like shapes.
2. Toss zucchini noodles with pesto sauce.
3. Add halved cherry tomatoes and toasted pine nuts.
4. Sprinkle with Parmesan cheese before serving.

Chicken and Vegetable Stir-Fry

Ingredients:

- Boneless, skinless chicken breast
- Soy sauce
- Ginger
- Garlic
- Broccoli florets

- Bell peppers
- Snap peas
- Brown rice

Instructions:

1. Cut chicken into thin strips and marinate in soy sauce, minced ginger, and minced garlic.
2. In a hot skillet, stir-fry the chicken until cooked.
3. Add broccoli, bell peppers, and snap peas.
4. Continue stir-frying until vegetables are tender.
5. Serve over cooked brown rice for a wholesome stir-fry.

Sweet Potato and Chickpea Curry

Ingredients:

- Sweet potatoes, peeled and cubed
- Chickpeas
- Coconut milk
- Curry paste
- Onion
- Garlic
- Spinach

Instructions:

1. In a pot, sauté diced onion and minced garlic.

2. Add sweet potato cubes, chickpeas, coconut milk, and curry paste.

3. Simmer until sweet potatoes are tender.

4. Stir in fresh spinach and let it wilt.

5. Serve this flavorful curry over rice or with naan bread.

Caesar Salad with Grilled Shrimp

Ingredients:

- Romaine lettuce
- Grilled shrimp
- Caesar dressing
- Croutons
- Grated Parmesan cheese

Instructions:

1. Toss crisp Romaine lettuce with grilled shrimp.

2. Drizzle with Caesar dressing.

3. Sprinkle croutons and grated Parmesan cheese on top.

4. Enjoy this satisfying and protein-packed Caesar salad.

Hummus and Veggie Wrap

Ingredients:

- Whole wheat tortillas
- Hummus
- Sliced cucumber
- Sliced red bell pepper
- Sliced avocado
- Baby spinach

Instructions:

1. Spread a generous layer of hummus on a whole wheat tortilla.
2. Layer on sliced cucumber, red bell pepper, sliced avocado, and baby spinach.
3. Roll up the tortilla, slice, and savor the delightful combination of flavors.

Cucumber and Feta Salad

Ingredients:

- Sliced cucumbers
- Crumbled feta cheese
- Cherry tomatoes
- Red onion rings
- Kalamata olives
- Greek dressing
- Fresh dill

Instructions:

1. Combine sliced cucumbers, crumbled feta cheese, cherry tomatoes, red onion rings, and Kalamata olives.
2. Drizzle with Greek dressing and garnish with fresh dill.
3. Delight in this refreshing cucumber and feta salad.

Spinach and Mushroom Quesadilla

Ingredients:

- Whole wheat tortillas

- Spinach leaves

- Sliced mushrooms

- Shredded low-fat cheese

- Olive oil

- Garlic

- Cumin

- Salt and pepper

Instructions:

1. Sauté sliced mushrooms and minced garlic in a bit of olive oil.
2. Season with cumin, salt, and pepper.
3. Place a whole wheat tortilla in a pan.
4. Layer with spinach leaves, sautéed mushrooms, and shredded low-fat cheese.
5. Top with another tortilla.
6. Cook until the quesadilla is golden and the cheese is melted.
7. Slice into wedges and enjoy this savory treat.

Couscous and Veggie Bowl

Ingredients:

- Couscous
- Mixed vegetables (zucchini, bell peppers, cherry tomatoes)
- Olive oil
- Lemon juice
- Fresh herbs (parsley, mint)
- Salt and pepper

Instructions:

1. Cook couscous according to package instructions.
2. Grill or roast mixed vegetables with olive oil.
3. Toss cooked couscous and vegetables together.
4. Drizzle with lemon juice and garnish with fresh herbs.
5. Savor this flavorful couscous and veggie bowl.

Tomato Basil Soup

Ingredients:

- Ripe tomatoes

- Onion

- Garlic

- Vegetable broth

- Fresh basil

- Olive oil

- Salt and pepper

Instructions:

1. Roast or grill ripe tomatoes, onion, and garlic with a drizzle of olive oil.
2. Blend the roasted ingredients with vegetable broth and fresh basil.
3. Season with salt and pepper.
4. Heat the soup and serve with a garnish of fresh basil.

Chapter 4: Dinner Recipes

In this chapter, we'll explore a diverse selection of delicious and wholesome dinner recipes that are perfect for your low-calorie meal prep journey. These recipes are designed to be both nutritious and flavorful, ensuring you enjoy every bite while maintaining your health goals. Let's dive into these delectable dishes!

Baked Salmon with Asparagus

Ingredients:

- 4 salmon fillets
- 1 bunch of asparagus
- 2 tablespoons olive oil
- 2 cloves of garlic, minced
- 1 lemon, sliced
- Salt and pepper to taste

Instructions:

1. Preheat your oven to 375°F (190°C).

2. Place the salmon fillets and asparagus on a baking sheet.

3. Drizzle olive oil over them, then sprinkle with minced garlic, salt, and pepper.

4. Lay lemon slices on top.

5. Bake for 15-20 minutes, or until the salmon flakes easily with a fork.

Spaghetti Squash with Marinara

Ingredients:

- 1 spaghetti squash
- 2 cups marinara sauce
- 1/2 cup grated Parmesan cheese
- Fresh basil leaves for garnish

Instructions:

1. Preheat the oven to 375°F (190°C).

2. Cut the spaghetti squash in half and scoop out the seeds.

3. Place the halves face down on a baking sheet and bake for 30-40 minutes.

4. Scrape the cooked squash into strands with a fork.

5. Heat the marinara sauce and serve over the spaghetti squash.

6. Top with grated Parmesan cheese and fresh basil.

Teriyaki Chicken with Broccoli

Ingredients:

- 2 boneless, skinless chicken breasts
- 1 cup broccoli florets
- 1/4 cup teriyaki sauce
- 2 tablespoons sesame seeds
- Cooked brown rice for serving

Instructions:

1. Cut chicken into bite-sized pieces and cook in a pan until no longer pink.

2. Add broccoli and cook until tender-crisp.

3. Pour teriyaki sauce over the chicken and broccoli.

4. Serve over brown rice and sprinkle with sesame seeds.

Stuffed Bell Peppers

Ingredients:

- 4 large bell peppers
- 1 pound lean ground turkey
- 1 cup cooked brown rice
- 1 cup marinara sauce
- 1/2 cup shredded mozzarella cheese
- Salt and pepper to taste

Instructions:

1. Cut the tops off the bell peppers and remove seeds and membranes.
2. In a skillet, brown ground turkey and season with salt and pepper.
3. Stir in cooked rice and marinara sauce.
4. Stuff the bell peppers with the mixture.
5. Sprinkle with mozzarella cheese.
6. Bake at 350°F (175°C) for 25-30 minutes.

Eggplant Parmesan

Ingredients:

- 1 large eggplant, sliced
- 1 cup whole-wheat breadcrumbs
- 1 cup marinara sauce
- 1 cup part-skim mozzarella cheese
- 1/4 cup grated Parmesan cheese
- Fresh basil leaves for garnish

Instructions:

1. Preheat your oven to 375°F (190°C).
2. Dip eggplant slices in egg, then coat with breadcrumbs.
3. Place the slices on a baking sheet and bake for 20-25 minutes.
4. In a baking dish, layer marinara sauce, eggplant slices, and cheese.
5. Repeat the layers and top with Parmesan cheese.
6. Bake for 30 minutes, until bubbly and golden.
7. Garnish with fresh basil leaves.

Lemon Garlic Shrimp and Quinoa

Ingredients:

- 1 pound large shrimp, peeled and deveined
- 1 cup quinoa
- 2 cloves garlic, minced
- Juice of 1 lemon
- 2 tablespoons olive oil
- Fresh parsley for garnish
- Salt and pepper to taste

Instructions:

1. Cook quinoa according to package instructions.
2. In a pan, sauté garlic in olive oil.
3. Add shrimp, lemon juice, salt, and pepper.
4. Cook until shrimp turn pink.
5. Serve over cooked quinoa and garnish with fresh parsley.

Turkey and Sweet Potato Chili

Ingredients:

- 1 pound ground turkey

- 2 sweet potatoes, diced

- 1 can black beans, drained and rinsed

- 1 can diced tomatoes

- 1 onion, chopped

- 2 cloves garlic, minced

- 2 tablespoons chili powder

- Salt and pepper to taste

Instructions:

1. In a large pot, brown the ground turkey.

2. Add chopped onion and garlic, cook until softened.

3. Stir in sweet potatoes, black beans, diced tomatoes, and chili powder.

4. Season with salt and pepper.

5. Simmer until sweet potatoes are tender.

Beef and Broccoli Stir-Fry

Ingredients:

- 1 pound lean beef, thinly sliced

- 2 cups broccoli florets

- 1/4 cup low-sodium soy sauce

- 2 tablespoons honey

- 2 cloves garlic, minced

- 1 tablespoon cornstarch

- Cooked brown rice for serving

Instructions:

1. In a bowl, mix soy sauce, honey, garlic, and cornstarch.
2. Heat a pan, add beef and cook until browned.
3. Add broccoli and stir-fry until tender.
4. Pour the sauce over and simmer until thickened.
5. Serve over cooked brown rice.

Butternut Squash Soup

Ingredients:

- 1 butternut squash, peeled and diced

- 1 onion, chopped

- 2 cloves garlic, minced

- 4 cups low-sodium vegetable broth

- 1 teaspoon ground cinnamon

- Salt and pepper to taste

Instructions:

1. In a pot, sauté onions and garlic until soft.

2. Add butternut squash and vegetable broth.

3. Season with cinnamon, salt, and pepper.

4. Simmer until squash is tender.

5. Blend the soup until smooth.

Spinach and Feta Stuffed Chicken Breast

Ingredients:

- 4 boneless, skinless chicken breasts

- 2 cups fresh spinach

- 1/2 cup crumbled feta cheese

- 2 cloves garlic, minced

- 1 tablespoon olive oil

- Salt and pepper to taste

Instructions:

1. Preheat your oven to 375°F (190°C).

2. Slice a pocket into each chicken breast.

3. In a pan, sauté spinach and garlic in olive oil.

4. Stuff each chicken breast with the sautéed spinach and feta.

5. Bake for 25-30 minutes.

Black Bean and Corn Salad

Ingredients:

- 1 can black beans, drained and rinsed
- 1 cup corn kernels
- 1 red bell pepper, diced
- 1/4 cup red onion, chopped
- 2 tablespoons lime juice
- 2 tablespoons fresh cilantro, chopped
- Salt and pepper to taste

Instructions:

1. In a bowl, combine black beans, corn, red pepper, and red onion.

2. Drizzle lime juice over the mixture.

3. Season with salt, pepper, and cilantro.

4. Toss well and refrigerate before serving.

Grilled Portobello Mushrooms

Ingredients:

- 4 portobello mushrooms
- 2 tablespoons balsamic vinegar
- 2 cloves garlic, minced
- 2 tablespoons olive oil
- Fresh thyme leaves for garnish
- Salt and pepper to taste

Instructions:

1. Clean the mushrooms and remove the stems.
2. In a bowl, mix balsamic vinegar, garlic, and olive oil.
3. Brush the mixture over the mushrooms.
4. Grill for 5-7 minutes on each side.
5. Garnish with fresh thyme leaves.

Veggie Stir-Fried Rice

Ingredients:

- 2 cups cooked brown rice
- 1 cup mixed vegetables (e.g., carrots, peas, bell peppers)

- 2 eggs, beaten
- 2 tablespoons low-sodium soy sauce
- 1 tablespoon sesame oil
- Green onions for garnish
- Salt and pepper to taste

Instructions:

1. In a pan, scramble the eggs and set them aside.
2. Stir-fry the mixed vegetables until tender.
3. Add cooked brown rice to the pan.
4. Pour soy sauce and sesame oil over the rice.
5. Add the scrambled eggs.
6. Season with salt, pepper, and garnish with chopped green onions.

Baked Cod with Lemon Dill Sauce

Ingredients:

- 4 cod fillets
- 1 lemon, sliced
- 2 cloves garlic, minced
- 2 tablespoons fresh dill, chopped
- 2 tablespoons olive oil

- Salt and pepper to taste

Instructions:

1. Preheat your oven to 375°F (190°C).
2. Place the cod fillets on a baking sheet.
3. Drizzle with olive oil and sprinkle minced garlic, dill, salt, and pepper.
4. Lay lemon slices on top.
5. Bake for 15-20 minutes or until the cod flakes easily with a fork.

Cauliflower Fried Rice

Ingredients:

- 1 small head of cauliflower, grated
- 1 cup mixed vegetables (e.g., peas, carrots, corn)
- 2 eggs, beaten
- 2 tablespoons low-sodium soy sauce
- 1 tablespoon sesame oil
- Green onions for garnish
- Salt and pepper to taste

Instructions:

1. In a pan, scramble the eggs and set them aside.
2. Stir-fry the mixed vegetables and grated cauliflower until tender.
3. Add the scrambled eggs, soy sauce, and sesame oil.
4. Season with salt, pepper, and garnish with chopped green onions.

Chapter 5: Snacks and Appetizers

In this chapter, we explore a variety of scrumptious snacks and appetizers that not only tantalize your taste buds but also keep those calorie counts in check. These options are perfect for satisfying those midday cravings or serving as delightful starters for any meal. Let's dive into these delectable low-calorie creations.

Guacamole and Veggie Sticks

Ingredients:

- 2 ripe avocados
- 1 lime, juiced
- 1 small tomato, diced
- 1/2 red onion, finely chopped
- 1 clove garlic, minced
- Salt and pepper to taste
- Assorted veggie sticks (carrots, celery, bell peppers)

Instructions:

1. Mash avocados in a bowl and mix with lime juice.

2. Add diced tomato, chopped red onion, minced garlic, salt, and pepper.

3. Stir well and serve with colorful veggie sticks.

Sliced Cucumber with Hummus

Ingredients:

- 1 cucumber, thinly sliced

- 1/2 cup of your favorite hummus

Instructions:

1. Arrange the cucumber slices on a plate.

2. Dip them in hummus for a refreshing and satisfying snack.

Baked Sweet Potato Fries

Ingredients:

- 2 medium sweet potatoes, cut into thin strips

- 1 tablespoon olive oil

- Salt, pepper, and paprika to taste

Instructions:

1. Preheat your oven to 425°F (220°C).

2. Toss sweet potato strips in olive oil and season with salt, pepper, and paprika.

3. Spread them on a baking sheet and bake for 20-25 minutes, turning halfway.

Mixed Nuts

Ingredients:

- A handful of mixed nuts (almonds, walnuts, cashews)

Instructions:

1. Grab your favorite assortment of unsalted nuts for a protein-packed snack.

Greek Yogurt and Berries

Ingredients:

- 1 cup Greek yogurt

- Mixed berries (strawberries, blueberries, raspberries)

Instructions:

1. Spoon Greek yogurt into a bowl and top with a handful of fresh mixed berries.

Popcorn

Ingredients:

- 1/2 cup of popcorn kernels
- Olive oil spray
- Salt and nutritional yeast (optional)

Instructions:

1. Pop the popcorn kernels using an air popper or stovetop method.
2. Lightly spray with olive oil and season with salt and nutritional yeast for a cheesy flavor.

Edamame

Ingredients:

- 1 cup frozen edamame
- Sea salt

Instructions:

1. Boil or steam edamame according to package instructions.
2. Sprinkle with sea salt before serving.

Rice Cakes with Peanut Butter

Ingredients:

- Rice cakes
- Natural peanut butter (no added sugar)

Instructions:

1. Spread a thin layer of peanut butter on rice cakes for a satisfying crunch with a hint of sweetness.

Deviled Eggs

Ingredients:

- 6 hard-boiled eggs
- 2 tablespoons Greek yogurt
- Dijon mustard to taste
- Paprika for garnish

Instructions:

1. Slice hard-boiled eggs in half, remove yolks, and mash them with Greek yogurt and Dijon mustard.
2. Spoon the mixture back into the egg whites and garnish with paprika.

Salsa and Baked Tortilla Chips

Ingredients:

- Baked whole-grain tortilla chips
- Fresh salsa or homemade tomato salsa

Instructions:

1. Dip those baked chips into zesty salsa for a satisfying snack with a kick.

Cottage Cheese with Pineapple

Ingredients:

- Low-fat cottage cheese
- Pineapple chunks (fresh or canned in juice)

Instructions:

1. Top a bowl of cottage cheese with pineapple chunks for a protein-packed sweet and savory treat.

Spinach and Artichoke Dip

Ingredients:

- 1 cup low-fat Greek yogurt
- 1 cup chopped spinach (frozen or fresh)
- 1/2 cup chopped artichoke hearts (canned in water)
- 1/4 cup grated Parmesan cheese
- 1 clove garlic, minced
- Salt and pepper to taste

Instructions:

1. Mix all ingredients in a microwave-safe bowl.
2. Heat until warm and bubbly, stirring occasionally.
3. Serve with raw veggie sticks or whole-grain crackers.

Trail Mix

Ingredients:

- Almonds, walnuts, and a variety of dried fruits

Instructions:

1. Create your own custom mix of nuts and dried fruits for a convenient, energy-boosting snack.

Stuffed Mushrooms

Ingredients:

- Fresh mushrooms
- A mixture of sautéed spinach, garlic, and low-fat cheese

Instructions:

1. Remove mushroom stems and stuff with the sautéed spinach and cheese mixture.
2. Bake until mushrooms are tender.

Sliced Apple with Almond Butter

Ingredients:

- Sliced apples
- Almond butter (unsweetened)

Instructions:

1. Dip apple slices into almond butter for a satisfying blend of textures and flavors.

Chapter 6: Desserts

In this chapter, we've curated a delectable collection of dessert recipes that are not only satisfying but also mindful of your health goals. From fruity parfaits to chocolatey delights, you'll find a sweet treat for every occasion. Get ready to savor these guilt-free desserts that will leave your taste buds dancing.

Berry Parfait

Ingredients:

- 1 cup of mixed berries (strawberries, blueberries, raspberries)
- 1 cup of Greek yogurt
- 1 tablespoon of honey
- 1/4 cup of granola

Instructions:

1. In a glass or bowl, layer the mixed berries.
2. Add a spoonful of Greek yogurt on top of the berries.
3. Drizzle with honey.

4. Sprinkle granola over the yogurt.

5. Repeat the layers.

6. Finish with a drizzle of honey and a few extra berries on top.

Chocolate Banana Ice Cream

Ingredients:

- 2 ripe bananas, sliced and frozen
- 2 tablespoons of unsweetened cocoa powder
- 1/2 teaspoon of vanilla extract
- Optional: a pinch of sea salt

Instructions:

1. Place the frozen banana slices, cocoa powder, and vanilla extract in a blender or food processor.

2. Blend until smooth, scraping down the sides as needed.

3. Add a pinch of sea salt if desired.

4. Serve immediately for a soft-serve consistency or freeze for a firmer texture.

Baked Apple with Cinnamon

Ingredients:

- 2 apples, cored and sliced
- 1/2 teaspoon of ground cinnamon
- 1 tablespoon of honey
- 2 tablespoons of chopped nuts (e.g., almonds or walnuts)

Instructions:

1. Preheat your oven to 350°F (175°C).
2. Place the apple slices in a baking dish.
3. Sprinkle with cinnamon and drizzle with honey.
4. Bake for 20-25 minutes until the apples are tender.
5. Sprinkle with chopped nuts before serving.

Greek Yogurt Cheesecake

Ingredients:

- 1 cup of Greek yogurt
- 1/4 cup of cream cheese (reduced-fat, if desired)
- 2 tablespoons of honey
- 1/2 teaspoon of vanilla extract

Instructions:

1. In a bowl, mix Greek yogurt, cream cheese, honey, and vanilla extract until smooth.

2. Pour the mixture into small serving dishes.

3. Refrigerate for at least 2 hours.

4. Serve with a drizzle of honey or fresh berries.

Mango Sorbet

Ingredients:

- 2 ripe mangoes, peeled and cubed
- 2 tablespoons of lime juice
- 1/4 cup of water
- 2 tablespoons of honey

Instructions:

1. Place the mango cubes, lime juice, water, and honey in a blender.

2. Blend until smooth.

3. Pour the mixture into a shallow container and freeze for a few hours, stirring occasionally, until firm.

4. Serve in scoops and garnish with fresh mint leaves.

Dark Chocolate-Dipped Strawberries

Ingredients:

- 12 fresh strawberries
- 2 ounces of dark chocolate (70% cocoa or higher)

Instructions:

1. Wash and dry the strawberries, leaving the stems intact.
2. Melt the dark chocolate in a microwave-safe bowl, stirring every 30 seconds until smooth.
3. Dip each strawberry into the melted chocolate, letting the excess drip off.
4. Place on a parchment-lined tray and let the chocolate set in the refrigerator.

Mini Fruit Tarts

Ingredients:

- 6 mini whole wheat tart shells
- 1/2 cup of Greek yogurt
- Assorted fresh fruits (e.g., berries, kiwi, mandarin oranges)

- 1 tablespoon of honey

Instructions:

1. Fill each tart shell with Greek yogurt.
2. Top with a variety of fresh fruits.
3. Drizzle with honey for extra sweetness.
4. Serve immediately or refrigerate until ready to enjoy.

Almond and Coconut Bites

Ingredients:

- 1 cup of unsweetened shredded coconut
- 1/2 cup of almond meal
- 2 tablespoons of honey
- 1/2 teaspoon of almond extract
- A pinch of salt

Instructions:

1. In a bowl, combine shredded coconut and almond meal.
2. Add honey, almond extract, and a pinch of salt, mixing until the mixture sticks together.
3. Form small bites and refrigerate until set.

Vanilla Chia Seed Pudding

Ingredients:

- 1/4 cup of chia seeds
- 1 cup of unsweetened almond milk
- 1/2 teaspoon of vanilla extract
- 1 tablespoon of maple syrup (optional)

Instructions:

1. In a jar, combine chia seeds, almond milk, vanilla extract, and maple syrup.
2. Stir well, cover, and refrigerate overnight.
3. Serve with fresh berries or a drizzle of honey.

Mixed Berry Crisp

Ingredients:

- 2 cups of mixed berries (strawberries, blueberries, raspberries)
- 1/4 cup of rolled oats
- 2 tablespoons of almond meal
- 1 tablespoon of honey
- 1/2 teaspoon of cinnamon

Instructions:

1. Preheat your oven to 350°F (175°C).
2. In a bowl, toss the mixed berries with honey and cinnamon.
3. In a separate bowl, mix rolled oats and almond meal.
4. Place the berry mixture in a baking dish and sprinkle the oat mixture over the top.
5. Bake for 20-25 minutes or until the topping is golden brown.

Lemon Sorbet

Ingredients:

- 3 lemons, juiced and zested
- 1/2 cup of water
- 1/4 cup of honey

Instructions:

1. In a saucepan, combine lemon juice, lemon zest, water, and honey.
2. Heat over medium heat, stirring until honey dissolves.
3. Remove from heat and let it cool.

4. Pour the mixture into a container and freeze, stirring occasionally until it reaches a sorbet consistency.

Chocolate Protein Balls

Ingredients:

- 1 cup of chocolate protein powder
- 1/4 cup of almond butter
- 1/4 cup of unsweetened cocoa powder
- 2 tablespoons of honey
- 1/2 teaspoon of vanilla extract

Instructions:

1. In a bowl, combine chocolate protein powder, almond butter, cocoa powder, honey, and vanilla extract.
2. Mix until the ingredients come together.
3. Roll the mixture into small balls.
4. Refrigerate until firm.

Rice Pudding

Ingredients:

- 1/2 cup of Arborio rice
- 2 cups of unsweetened almond milk
- 1/4 cup of honey
- 1/2 teaspoon of vanilla extract
- A pinch of cinnamon

Instructions:

1. In a saucepan, combine rice, almond milk, honey, and vanilla extract.
2. Cook over low heat, stirring regularly, until the rice is tender and the mixture thickens.
3. Sprinkle with a pinch of cinnamon before serving.

Frozen Grapes

Ingredients:

- Fresh grapes (any variety)

Instructions:

1. Wash and dry the grapes.

2. Place them in a single layer on a baking sheet.

3. Freeze until solid.

4. Enjoy these icy, sweet treats straight from the freezer.

Pumpkin Pie Bites

Ingredients:

- 1/2 cup of pumpkin puree
- 1/4 cup of almond meal
- 1/4 cup of rolled oats
- 2 tablespoons of honey
- 1/2 teaspoon of pumpkin pie spice

Instructions:

1. In a bowl, mix pumpkin puree, almond meal, rolled oats, honey, and pumpkin pie spice.

2. Form the mixture into bite-sized balls.

3. Refrigerate until set.

Chapter 7: Smoothies

Whether you're looking for a refreshing start to your morning or a healthy afternoon snack, this chapter offers unique and delicious smoothie recipes to tantalize your taste buds. Packed with fresh fruits, vegetables, and a touch of creativity, these smoothies are a delightful way to boost your energy and nourish your body.

Green Detox Smoothie

Ingredients:

- 1 cup kale
- 1/2 cucumber
- 1 green apple
- 1/2 lemon (juiced)
- 1 cup water
- 1/2 cup ice

Instructions:

1. Blend kale, cucumber, and green apple until smooth.
2. Add lemon juice, water, and ice. Blend until creamy.

Berry Blast Smoothie

Ingredients:

- 1 cup mixed berries (strawberries, blueberries, raspberries)
- 1/2 cup Greek yogurt
- 1 banana
- 1/2 cup almond milk
- 1 tablespoon honey

Instructions:

1. Combine mixed berries, Greek yogurt, banana, almond milk, and honey.
2. Blend until you achieve a smooth consistency.

Tropical Paradise Smoothie

Ingredients:

- 1 cup pineapple chunks
- 1/2 banana
- 1/2 cup coconut milk
- 1/4 cup orange juice
- 1/2 cup ice

Instructions:

1. Blend pineapple, banana, coconut milk, and orange juice.
2. Add ice and blend until it's nice and frosty.

Peanut Butter and Banana Smoothie

Ingredients:

- 1 banana
- 2 tablespoons peanut butter
- 1 cup almond milk
- 1 tablespoon honey
- 1/2 cup ice

Instructions:

1. Combine banana, peanut butter, almond milk, honey, and ice.
2. Blend until you have a creamy and delightful concoction.

Spinach and Pineapple Smoothie

Ingredients:

- 2 cups spinach
- 1 cup pineapple chunks
- 1/2 cup coconut water
- 1/2 banana
- 1/2 cup ice

Instructions:

1. Blend spinach, pineapple, coconut water, and banana.
2. Add ice and blend until your smoothie is perfectly green and refreshingly tropical.

Blueberry Almond Smoothie

Ingredients:

- 1 cup blueberries
- 1/4 cup almonds
- 1 cup almond milk
- 1/2 banana
- 1 tablespoon honey

- 1/2 cup ice

Instructions:

1. Combine blueberries, almonds, almond milk, banana, honey, and ice in a blender.
2. Blend until it reaches a smooth and vibrant blue hue.

Chocolate Protein Shake

Ingredients:

- 1 scoop chocolate protein powder
- 1 cup almond milk
- 1 banana
- 2 tablespoons cocoa powder
- 1/2 cup ice

Instructions:

1. Blend chocolate protein powder, almond milk, banana, cocoa powder, and ice until rich and chocolaty.

Kale and Mango Smoothie

Ingredients:

- 1 cup kale
- 1/2 cup mango chunks
- 1/2 cup orange juice
- 1/2 cup Greek yogurt
- 1/2 cup ice

Instructions:

1. Blend kale, mango, orange juice, Greek yogurt, and ice until it's vibrant and smooth.

Strawberry Kiwi Smoothie

Ingredients:

- 1 cup strawberries
- 2 kiwis, peeled
- 1/2 cup Greek yogurt
- 1/2 cup orange juice
- 1/2 cup ice

Instructions:

1. Combine strawberries, kiwis, Greek yogurt, orange juice, and ice.

2. Blend until you have a delightful pink concoction.

Oatmeal Cookie Smoothie

Ingredients:

- 1/2 cup rolled oats
- 1/2 banana
- 1/4 cup almond butter
- 1/2 teaspoon cinnamon
- 1 cup almond milk
- 1/2 cup ice

Instructions:

1. Blend rolled oats, banana, almond butter, cinnamon, almond milk, and ice until it's like an oatmeal cookie in a glass.

Cucumber and Mint Smoothie

Ingredients:

- 1/2 cucumber
- 1/2 cup mint leaves
- 1/2 lemon (juiced)
- 1 cup coconut water
- 1/2 cup ice

Instructions:

1. Blend cucumber, mint leaves, lemon juice, coconut water, and ice until it's fresh and rejuvenating.

Carrot Cake Smoothie

Ingredients:

- 1 cup grated carrots
- 1/2 cup Greek yogurt
- 1/4 cup rolled oats
- 1/2 teaspoon cinnamon
- 1 tablespoon honey
- 1/2 cup ice

Instructions:

1. Combine grated carrots, Greek yogurt, rolled oats, cinnamon, honey, and ice.

2. Blend until it's reminiscent of a carrot cake.

Watermelon Cucumber Cooler

Ingredients:

- 1 cup watermelon chunks

- 1/2 cucumber

- 1/2 lime (juiced)

- 1/2 cup coconut water

- 1/2 cup ice

Instructions:

1. Blend watermelon, cucumber, lime juice, coconut water, and ice until it's a hydrating and refreshing cooler.

Raspberry Almond Smoothie

Ingredients:

- 1 cup raspberries

- 1/4 cup almonds

- 1 cup almond milk

- 1/2 banana

- 1 tablespoon honey

- 1/2 cup ice

Instructions:

1. Combine raspberries, almonds, almond milk, banana, honey, and ice.

2. Blend until it's a delightful pink hue with a nutty twist.

Avocado and Spinach Smoothie

Ingredients:

- 1/2 avocado

- 2 cups spinach

- 1/2 cup coconut water

- 1/2 cup Greek yogurt

- 1/2 cup ice

Instructions:

1. Blend avocado, spinach, coconut water, Greek yogurt, and ice until it's creamy and packed with greens.

CONCLUSION

As we approach the final chapter of our low-calorie meal prep adventure, it's time to reflect on the journey you've embarked upon. This concluding chapter is not a farewell but a celebration of your newfound knowledge and skills in the world of healthy eating.

Throughout this book, you've delved into the art of low-calorie meal preparation, discovering an array of delicious recipes and innovative techniques that have empowered you to take control of your nutrition. In this concluding chapter, we'll wrap up our exploration by offering some key insights, tips, and resources to ensure your success well beyond the last page.

Tips for Long-Term Success

- **Sustainability is key:** We'll discuss strategies for maintaining your low-calorie meal plan over the long haul. Learn how to make this a lifestyle, not just a temporary fix.

- **Meal prepping wisdom:** Discover the best practices for efficient meal prepping. Save time and effort while keeping your meals exciting and nutritious.
- **Staying on track:** We'll delve into ways to stay motivated and overcome common hurdles. Maintaining a healthy eating regimen can be challenging, but we'll equip you with the tools to persevere.

Staying Motivated

- **Finding your why:** Explore the importance of identifying your personal motivations for choosing a low-calorie lifestyle. Your "why" is your driving force.
- **Celebrating victories:** Learn the significance of celebrating small and large milestones on your journey. Recognizing your achievements keeps you inspired.
- **Building a support system:** Discover the power of a supportive community. Surround yourself with

like-minded individuals who can encourage and motivate you.

This Chapter is your gateway to a future filled with delicious, health-conscious meals and newfound knowledge. It's not a conclusion but the beginning of a lifelong journey towards a healthier you. Keep the spirit of curiosity and determination alive as you explore the world of low-calorie cuisine.